My Mediterranean Daily Recipes

Easy & Healthy Mediterranean Recipes To Make Unforgettable First Courses

Dan Peterson

TABLE OF CONTENT

Bean Balls with Marinara... 5
Confetti Couscous.. 7
Lemon-Herbs Orzo.. 8
Mediterranean Orzo and Vegetables Pilaf......................10
Lentils and Bulgur Wheat and Browned Onions...........11
Quick Spanish Rice.. 13
Rustic Lentil and Basmati Rice Pilaf.................................14
Creamy Polenta with Parmesan Cheese......................... 16
Bean and Toasted Pita Salad..17
Beans and Spinach Mediterranean Salad....................... 19
Chickpea Fried Eggplant Salad.. 21
Scorched Beet Almond Salad...25
Sweet Nut Winter Squash Salad.. 27
Tomato Mix Salad...29
Tomato-Burrata Mix Salad..30
Loaded Caesar Salad with Crunchy Chickpeas.......... 32
Coleslaw Worth A Second Helping....................................34
Romaine Lettuce and Radicchios Mix.............................. 35
Asparagus and Smoked Salmon Salad........................... 36
Shrimp Cobb Salad... 38
Classic Niçoise Salad.. 40

Algerian Carrot Slaw.. *42*
Tabbouleh (Lebanese Parsley and Bulgur Salad)....................... *43*
Cucumber and Red Onion Salad.. *44*
Mediterranean Quinoa Salad... *45*
French Potato Dijon Herb Salad..*47*
Green Bean Cilantro Salad... *49*
Italian Panzanella Mix Salad...*51*
Mackerel-Fennel-Apple Salad...*53*
Moroccan Carrot Salad... *55*
Algerian Mix Salad..*57*
Asparagus Mix Salad.. *58*
Brussels Pecorino Pine Salad... *60*
Cauliflower Chermoula Salad... *61*
Cherry Tomato Mix Salad... *63*
Classic Greek Salad.. *65*
Crunchy Mushroom Salad.. *67*
Cucumber Sesame-Lemon Salad... *68*
Cut Up Salad... *69*
Fattoush.. *71*
Toast with Smoked Salmon, Herbed Cream Cheese, and Greens 73
Crab Melt with Avocado and Egg... *75*
Tomato Cucumber Avocado Salad...*77*
Healthy Broccoli Salad.. *78*
Avocado Lime Shrimp Salad.. *79*

Grilled Mahi-Mahi with Jicama Slaw..........80
Mediterranean Chicken Salad..........82
Shrimp Salad Cocktails..........84
Garlic Chive Cauliflower Mash..........86
Beet Greens with Pine Nuts Goat Cheese..........87
Kale Slaw and Strawberry Salad + Poppyseed Dressing..........88
Spring Greek Salad..........90
Panzanella..........91
Tuscan Tuna Salad..........93
Mediterranean Chopped Salad..........94
Green Bean and Potato Salad..........96
Shrimp Salad..........98
Warm Potato Salad..........99
Summer Rainbow Salad..........100
Arugula and White Bean Salad..........101
Fennel and Orange Salad..........102
Balsamic Asparagus..........103
Lime Cucumber Mix..........104
Walnuts Cucumber Mix..........105
Cheesy Beet Salad..........106
Rosemary Beets..........107
Squash and Tomatoes Mix..........108

© **Copyright 2021 - All rights reserved.**

The content contained within this book may not be reproduced, duplicated or transmitted without direct written permission from the author or the publisher.

Under no circumstances will any blame or legal responsibility be held against the publisher, or author, for any damages, reparation, or monetary loss due to the information contained within this book. Either directly or indirectly.

Legal Notice:

This book is copyright protected. This book is only for personal use. You cannot amend, distribute, sell, use, quote or paraphrase any part, or the content within this book, without the consent of the author or publisher.

Disclaimer Notice:

Please note the information contained within this document is for educational and entertainment purposes only. All effort has been executed to present accurate, up to date, and reliable, complete information. No warranties of any kind are declared or implied. Readers acknowledge that the author is not engaging in the rendering of legal, financial, medical or professional advice. The content within this book has been derived from various sources. Please consult a licensed professional before attempting any techniques outlined in this book.

By reading this document, the reader agrees that under no circumstances is the author responsible for any losses, direct or indirect, which are incurred as a result of the use of information contained within this document, including, but not limited to, — errors, omissions, or inaccuracies.

Bean Balls with Marinara

Preparation time: 15 minutes

Cooking time: 30 minutes

Servings: 2-4

INGREDIENTS:
- Bean Balls:
- 1 tablespoon extra-virgin olive oil
- ½ yellow onion, minced
- 1 teaspoon fennel seeds
- 2 teaspoons dried oregano
- ½ teaspoon crushed red pepper flakes
- 1 teaspoon garlic powder
- 1 (15-ounce / 425-g) can white beans (cannellini or navy), drained and rinsed
- ½ cup whole-grain bread crumbs
- Sea salt and ground black pepper, to taste
- Marinara:
- 1 tablespoon extra-virgin olive oil
- 3 garlic cloves, minced
- Handful basil leaves
- 1 (28-ounce / 794-g) can chopped tomatoes with juice reserved
- Sea salt, to taste

DIRECTIONS:
1. Preheat the oven to 350°F (180°C). Line a baking sheet with parchment paper. Heat the olive oil in a nonstick skillet over medium heat until shimmering.
2. Add the onion and sauté for 5 minutes or until translucent. Sprinkle with fennel seeds, oregano, red pepper flakes, and

garlic powder, then cook for 1 minute or until aromatic.
3. Pour the sautéed mixture in a food processor and add the beans and bread crumbs. Sprinkle with salt and ground black pepper, then pulse to combine well and the mixture holds together.
4. Shape the mixture into balls with a 2-ounce (57-g) cookie scoop, then arrange the balls on the baking sheet.
5. Bake in the preheated oven for 30 minutes or until lightly browned. Flip the balls halfway through the cooking time.
6. While baking the bean balls, heat the olive oil in a saucepan over medium-high heat until shimmering. Add the garlic and basil and sauté for 2 minutes or until fragrant.
7. Fold in the tomatoes and juice. Bring to a boil. Reduce the heat to low. Put the lid on and simmer for 15 minutes. Sprinkle with salt.
8. Transfer the bean balls on a large plate and baste with marinara before serving.

NUTRITION: Calories: 351 Fat: 16.4g Protein: 11.5g Carbs: 42.9g

Confetti Couscous

Preparation time : 5 minutes

Cooking time: 20 minutes

Servings: 4-6

INGREDIENTS:
- 3 tablespoons olive oil
- 1 large chopped onion
- 1 cup fresh peas
- 2 carrots, chopped
- ½ cup golden raisins
- 1 teaspoon salt
- 2 cups vegetable broth
- 2 cups couscous

DIRECTIONS:
1. Add the olive oil, onions, peas, raisins, and carrots to a skillet over medium heat. Allow to cook for 5 minutes, stirring occasionally, or until the vegetables start to soften.
2. Season with salt and pour in the vegetable broth while whisking. Bring it to a boil for about 5 minutes. Fold in the couscous and stir to combine.
3. Reduce the heat to low and cook covered for about 10 minutes, or until the couscous has absorbed the liquid completely. Using a fork to fluff the couscous and serve while warm.

NUTRITION: Calories: 515 Fat: 12.3g Carbs: 92.3g Protein: 14.2g

Lemon-Herbs Orzo

Preparation time: 15 minutes

Cooking time: 10 minutes

Servings: 4

INGREDIENTS:
- Orzo:
- 2 cups orzo
- ½ cup fresh basil, finely chopped
- 2 tablespoons lemon zest
- ½ cup fresh parsley, finely chopped
- Dressing:
- ½ cup extra-virgin olive oil
- 1/3 cup lemon juice
- 1 teaspoon salt
- ½ teaspoon freshly ground black pepper

DIRECTIONS:
1. Put the orzo in a large saucepan of boiling water and allow to cook for 6 minutes. Drain the orzo in a sieve and rinse well under cold running water. Set aside to cool completely.
2. When cooled, place the orzo in a large bowl. Mix in the basil, lemon zest, and parsley. Set aside.
3. Make the dressing: In a separate bowl, combine the olive oil, lemon juice, salt, and pepper. Stir to incorporate.
4. Pour the dressing into the bowl of orzo mixture and toss gently until everything is well combined. Serve immediately, or refrigerate for later.

NUTRITION: Calories: 570 Fat: 29.3g Carbs: 65.1g Protein: 11.2g

Mediterranean Orzo and Vegetables Pilaf

Preparation time: 15 minutes

Cooking time: 10 minutes

Servings: 6

INGREDIENTS:
- 2 cups orzo
- 1 cup Kalamata olives
- 1 pint (2 cups) cherry tomatoes, cut in half
- ½ cup fresh basil, finely chopped
- Dressing:
- ½ cup extra-virgin olive oil
- 1/3 cup balsamic vinegar
- 1 teaspoon salt
- ½ teaspoon freshly ground black pepper

DIRECTIONS:
1. Put the orzo in a large pot of boiling water and allow to cook for 6 minutes. Drain the orzo in a sieve and rinse well under cold running water. Set aside to cool completely.
2. When cooled, place the orzo in a large bowl. Add the olives, tomatoes, and basil. Toss well.
3. Mix together the olive oil, vinegar, pepper, and salt in a separate bowl. Pour the dressing into the bowl of orzo and vegetables.
4. Toss gently to mix them thoroughly. Serve chilled or at room temperature.

NUTRITION: Calories: 480 Fat: 28.3g Carbs: 48.2g Protein: 8.1g

Lentils and Bulgur Wheat and Browned Onions

Preparation time: 15 minutes

Cooking time: 35 minutes

Servings: 6

INGREDIENTS:
- ½ cup olive oil
- 4 large chopped onions
- 2 teaspoons salt, divided
- 2 cups brown lentils, picked over and rinsed
- 6 cups water
- 1 cup bulgur wheat
- 1 teaspoon freshly ground black pepper

DIRECTIONS:
1. Heat the olive oil in a saucepan over medium heat. Add the onions and sauté for 3 to 4 minutes until the edges are lightly browned.
2. Season with 1 teaspoon of salt. Reserve half of the cooked onions on a platter for later use.
3. Add the remaining salt, lentils, and water to the remaining onions in the saucepan. Stir to combine and cook covered for about 20 to 25 minutes, stirring occasionally.
4. Fold in the bulgur wheat and sprinkle with the black pepper. Give it a good stir and cook for 5 minutes more. Using a fork to fluff the mixture, cover, and allow to sit for 5 minutes.

5. Remove from the saucepan to six serving plates. Serve topped with the reserved cooked onions.

NUTRITION: Calories: 485 Fat: 20.4g Carbs: 59.5g Protein: 20.1g

Quick Spanish Rice

Preparation time: 10 minutes

Cooking time: 15 minutes

Servings: 4

INGREDIENTS:
- 2 tablespoons olive oil
- 1 medium onion, finely chopped
- 1 large tomato, finely diced
- 1 teaspoon smoked paprika
- 2 tablespoons tomato paste
- 1½ cups basmati rice
- 1 teaspoon salt
- 3 cups water

DIRECTIONS:
1. Heat the olive oil in a saucepan over medium heat. Add the onions and tomato and sauté for about 3 minutes until softened.
2. Add the paprika, tomato paste, basmati rice, and salt. Stir the mixture for 1 minute and slowly pour in the water.
3. Reduce the heat to low and allow to simmer covered for 12 minutes, stirring constantly. Remove from the heat and let it rest in the saucepan for 3 minutes. Divide the rice evenly among four serving bowls and serve.

NUTRITION: Calories: 331 Fat: 7.3g Carbs: 59.8g Protein: 6.1g

Rustic Lentil and Basmati Rice Pilaf

Preparation time: 15 minutes

Cooking time: 50 minutes

Servings: 6

INGREDIENTS:
- ¼ cup olive oil
- 1 large onion, chopped
- 1 teaspoon ground cumin
- 1 teaspoon salt
- 6 cups water
- 2 cups brown lentils, picked over and rinsed
- 1 cup basmati rice

DIRECTIONS:
1. Heat the olive oil in a saucepan over medium heat. Add the onions and cook for about 4 minutes until the onions are a medium golden color.
2. Turn the heat to high and add the cumin, salt, and water. Allow the mixture to boil for about 3 minutes until heated through.
3. Reduce the heat to medium-low and add the brown lentils. Allow to simmer covered for about 20 minutes until tender, stirring occasionally.
4. Add the basmati rice and stir well. Cook for 20 minutes until the rice has absorbed the liquid completely.
5. Using a fork to fluff the rice, cover, and let stand for 5 minutes. Transfer to plates and

serve hot.
NUTRITION: Calories: 400 Fat: 11.3g Carbs: 59.7g Protein: 18.4g

Creamy Polenta with Parmesan Cheese

Preparation time: 15 minutes

Cooking time: 25 minutes

Servings: 4

INGREDIENTS:
- 3 tablespoons olive oil
- 1 tablespoon garlic, finely chopped
- 1 teaspoon salt
- 4 cups water
- 1 cup polenta
- ¾ cup Parmesan cheese, divided

DIRECTIONS:
1. In a large saucepan, heat the olive oil over medium heat. Cook the garlic for 2 minutes until fragrant. Season with 1 teaspoon salt.
2. Pour in the water and bring it to a rapid boil. Fold in the polenta and stir for 3 minutes until it begins to thicken.
3. Reduce the heat to low, cover, and allow to simmer covered for about 20 minutes, whisking constantly.
4. Add the ½ cup of the Parmesan cheese and stir to combine. Divide the polenta into four serving bowls and serve sprinkled with remaining cheese.

NUTRITION: Calories: 300 Fat: 15.8g Carbs: 27.5g Protein: 8.7g

Bean and Toasted Pita Salad

Preparation time: 15 minutes

Cooking time: 6 minutes

Servings: 4

INGREDIENTS:
- 3 tbsp chopped fresh mint
- 3 tbsp chopped fresh parsley
- 1 cup crumbled feta cheese
- 1 cup sliced romaine lettuce
- ½ cucumber, peeled and sliced
- 1 cup diced plum tomatoes
- 2 cups cooked pinto beans, well drained and slightly warmed
- Pepper to taste
- 3 tbsp extra virgin olive oil
- 2 tbsp ground toasted cumin seeds
- 2 tbsp fresh lemon juice
- 1/8 tsp salt
- 2 cloves garlic, peeled
- 2 6-inch whole wheat pita bread, cut or torn into bite-sized pieces

DIRECTIONS:
1. In large baking sheet, spread torn pita bread and bake in a preheated 400F oven for 6 minutes. With the back of a knife, mash garlic and salt until paste like. Add into a medium bowl.
2. Whisk in ground cumin and lemon juice. In a steady and slow stream, pour oil as you whisk continuously. Season with pepper.

3. In a large salad bowl, mix cucumber, tomatoes and beans. Pour in dressing, toss to coat well. Add mint, parsley, feta, lettuce and toasted pita, toss to mix once again and serve.

NUTRITION: Calories: 427 Protein: 17.7g Carbs: 47.3g Fat: 20.4g

Beans and Spinach Mediterranean Salad

Preparation time: 15 minutes

Cooking time: 15 minutes

Servings: 4

INGREDIENTS:
- 1 can (14 ounces) water-packed artichoke hearts, rinsed, drained and quartered
- 1 can (14-1/2 ounces) no-salt-added diced tomatoes, undrained
- 1 can (15 ounces) cannellini beans, rinsed and drained
- 1 small onion, chopped
- 1 tablespoon olive oil
- 1/4 teaspoon pepper
- 1/4 teaspoon salt
- 1/8 teaspoon crushed red pepper flakes
- 2 garlic cloves, minced
- 2 tablespoons Worcestershire sauce
- 6 ounces fresh baby spinach (about 8 cups)
- Additional olive oil, optional

DIRECTIONS:
1. Place a saucepan on medium high fire and heat for a minute. Add oil and heat for 2 minutes. Stir in onion and sauté for 4 minutes. Add garlic and sauté for another minute.
2. Stir in seasonings, Worcestershire sauce, and tomatoes. Cook for 5 minutes while stirring continuously until sauce is reduced.

3. Stir in spinach, artichoke hearts, and beans. Sauté for 3 minutes until spinach is wilted and other ingredients are heated through. Serve and enjoy.

NUTRITION: Calories: 187 Protein: 8.0g Carbs: 30.0g Fat: 4.0g

Chickpea Fried Eggplant Salad

Preparation time: 15 minutes

Cooking time: 12 minutes

Servings: 4

INGREDIENTS:
- 1 cup chopped dill
- 1 cup chopped parsley
- 1 cup cooked or canned chickpeas, drained
- 1 large eggplant, thinly sliced (no more than 1/4 inch in thickness)
- 1 small red onion, sliced in 1/2 moons
- 1/2 English cucumber, diced
- 3 Roma tomatoes, diced
- 3 tbsp Za'atar spice, divided
- oil for frying, preferably extra virgin olive oil
- Salt
- Garlic Vinaigrette Ingredients:
- 1 large lime, juice of
- 1/3 cup extra virgin olive oil
- 1-2 garlic cloves, minced
- Salt & Pepper to taste

DIRECTIONS:
1. On a baking sheet, spread out sliced eggplant and season with salt generously. Let it sit for 30 minutes. Then pat dry with paper towel.
2. Place a small pot on medium high fire and fill halfway with oil. Heat oil for 5 minutes. Fry eggplant in batches until golden brown,

around 3 minutes per side.
3. Place cooked eggplants on a paper towel lined plate. Once eggplants have cooled, assemble the eggplant on a serving dish. Sprinkle with 1 tbsp of Za'atar.
4. Mix dill, parsley, red onions, chickpeas, cucumbers, and tomatoes in a large salad bowl. Sprinkle remaining Za'atar and gently toss to mix.
5. Whisk well the vinaigrette ingredients in a small bowl. Drizzle 2 tbsp of the dressing over the fried eggplant. Add remaining dressing over the chickpea salad and mix.
6. Add the chickpea salad to the serving dish with the fried eggplant. Serve and enjoy.

NUTRITION: Calories: 642 Protein: 16.6g Carbs: 25.9g Fat: 44.0g

SALAD RECIPES

159. Radish-Fava Salad

Preparation time: 15 minutes

Cooking time: 5 minutes

Servings: 4-6

INGREDIENTS:
- ¼ cup chopped fresh basil
- ¼ cup extra-virgin olive oil
- ¼ teaspoon ground coriander
- ¼ teaspoon pepper
- ½ teaspoon salt
- 10 radishes, trimmed, halved, and sliced thin
- 1½ ounces (1½ cups) pea shoots
- 2 garlic cloves, minced
- 3 pounds fava beans, shelled (3 cups)
- 3 tablespoons lemon juice

DIRECTIONS:
1. Bring 4 quarts water to boil in large pot on high heat. In the meantime, fill big container halfway with ice and water.
2. Put in fava beans to boiling water and cook for about sixty seconds. Drain fava beans, move to ice water, and allow to sit until chilled, approximately two minutes.
3. Move fava beans to triple layer of paper towels and dry well. Use a paring knife to make small cut along edge of each bean through waxy sheath, then gently squeeze sheath to release bean; discard sheath.
4. Beat lemon juice, garlic, salt, pepper, and coriander together in a big container.

Whisking continuously, slowly drizzle in oil.
5. Put in fava beans, radishes, pea shoots, and basil and gently toss to coat. Serve instantly.

NUTRITION: Calories: 158 Carbs: 13g Fat: 10g Protein: 4g

Scorched Beet Almond Salad

Preparation time: 15 minutes

Cooking time: 0 minutes

Servings : 4-6

INGREDIENTS:
- 2 blood oranges
- 2 ounces (2 cups) baby arugula
- 2 ounces ricotta salata cheese, shaved
- 2 pounds beets, trimmed
- 2 tablespoons extra-virgin olive oil
- 2 tablespoons sliced almonds, toasted
- 4 teaspoons sherry vinegar
- Salt and pepper

DIRECTIONS:
1. Place the oven rack in the center of the oven and pre-heat your oven to 400 degrees. Wrap each beet individually in aluminum foil and place in rimmed baking sheet.
2. Roast beets until it is easy to skewer the center of beets with foil removed, forty minutes to one hour.
3. Cautiously open foil packets and allow beets to sit until cool enough to handle. Cautiously rub off beet skins using a paper towel. Slice beets into ½-inch-thick wedges, and, if large, cut in half crosswise.
4. Beat vinegar, ¼ teaspoon salt, and ¼ teaspoon pepper together in a big container. Whisking continuously, slowly

drizzle in oil.
5. Put in beets, toss to coat, and allow to cool to room temperature, approximately twenty minutes.
6. Cut away peel and pith from oranges. Quarter oranges, then slice crosswise into ½-inch-thick pieces. Put in oranges and arugula to a container with beets and gently toss to coat.
7. Sprinkle with salt and pepper to taste. Move to serving platter and drizzle with ricotta salata and almonds. Serve.

NUTRITION: Calories: 275 Carbs: 22g Fat: 19g Protein: 5g

Sweet Nut Winter Squash Salad

Preparation time: 15 minutes
Cooking time : 0 minutes

Servings: 4-6

INGREDIENTS:
- ¼ cup extra-virgin olive oil
- 1/3 cup roasted, unsalted pepitas
- ½ cup pomegranate seeds
- ¾ cup fresh parsley leaves
- 1 small shallot, minced
- 1 teaspoon za'atar
- 2 tablespoons honey
- 2 tablespoons lemon juice
- 3 pounds butternut squash, peeled, seeded, and cut into ½-inch pieces (8 cups)
- Salt and pepper

DIRECTIONS:
1. Place oven rack to lowest position and pre-heat your oven to 450 degrees. Toss squash with 1 tablespoon oil and sprinkle with salt and pepper.
2. Arrange squash in one layer in rimmed baking sheet and roast until thoroughly browned and tender, 30 to 35 minutes, stirring halfway through roasting. Sprinkle squash with za'atar and allow to cool for about fifteen minutes.
3. Beat shallot, lemon juice, honey, and ¼ teaspoon salt together in a big container.

Whisking continuously, slowly drizzle in remaining 3 tablespoons oil.
4. Put in squash, parsley, and pepitas and gently toss to coat. Arrange salad on serving platter and drizzle with pomegranate seeds. Serve.

NUTRITION: Calories: 385 Carbs: 0g •Fat: 6g •Protein: 7g

Tomato Mix Salad

Preparation time: 15 minutes
Cooking time : 0 minutes

Servings: 6

INGREDIENTS:
- ¼ cup plain Greek yogurt
- 1 garlic clove, minced
- 1 scallion, sliced thin
- 1 tablespoon extra-virgin olive oil
- 1 tablespoon lemon juice
- 1 tablespoon minced fresh oregano
- 1 teaspoon ground cumin
- 2½ pounds ripe tomatoes, cored and cut into ½-inch-thick wedges
- 3 ounces feta cheese, crumbled (¾ cup)
- Salt and pepper

DIRECTIONS:
1. Toss tomatoes with ½ teaspoon salt and allow to drain using a colander set over bowl for fifteen to twenty minutes.
2. Microwave oil, garlic, and cumin in a container until aromatic, approximately half a minute; allow to cool slightly. Move 1 tablespoon tomato liquid to big container; discard remaining liquid.
3. Beat in yogurt, lemon juice, scallion, oregano, and oil mixture until combined. Put in tomatoes and feta and gently toss to coat. Sprinkle with salt and pepper to taste. Serve.

NUTRITION: Calories: 60 Carbs: 0g Fat: 5g Protein: 0g

Tomato-Burrata Mix Salad

Preparation time: 15 minutes

Cooking time: 10 minutes

Servings: 4-6

INGREDIENTS:
- ½ cup chopped fresh basil
- 1 garlic clove, minced
- 1 shallot, halved and sliced thin
- 1½ pounds ripe tomatoes, cored and cut into 1-inch pieces
- 1½ tablespoons white balsamic vinegar
- 3 ounces rustic Italian bread, cut into 1-inch pieces (1 cup)
- 6 tablespoons extra-virgin olive oil
- 8 ounces burrata cheese, room temperature
- 8 ounces ripe cherry tomatoes, halved
- Salt and pepper

DIRECTIONS:
- Toss tomatoes with ¼ teaspoon salt and allow to drain using a colander for 30 minutes.
- Pulse bread using a food processor into large crumbs measuring between 1/8 and ¼ inch, approximately ten pulses.
- Mix crumbs, 2 tablespoons oil, pinch salt, and pinch pepper in 12-inch non-stick skillet. Cook on moderate heat, stirring frequently, until crumbs are crisp and golden, about 10 minutes.

- Clear center of skillet, put in garlic, and cook, mashing it into skillet, until aromatic, approximately half a minute. Stir garlic into crumbs. Move to plate and allow to cool slightly.
- Beat shallot, vinegar, and ¼ teaspoon salt together in a big container. Whisking continuously, slowly drizzle in remaining ¼ cup oil. Put in tomatoes and basil and gently toss to combine.
- Sprinkle with salt and pepper to taste and arrange on serving platter. Cut buratta into 1-inch pieces, collecting creamy liquid.
- Sprinkle burrata over tomatoes and drizzle with creamy liquid. Sprinkle with bread crumbs and serve instantly.

NUTRITION: Calories: 470 Carbs: 24g Fat: 32g Protein: 19g

Loaded Caesar Salad with Crunchy Chickpeas

Preparation Time: 5 minutes

Cooking Time: 20 minutes

Servings: 6

INGREDIENTS:
- For the chickpeas:
- 2 (15-ounce) cans chickpeas, drained and rinsed
- 2 tablespoons extra-virgin olive oil
- 1 teaspoon kosher salt
- 1 teaspoon garlic powder
- 1 teaspoon onion powder
- 1 teaspoon dried oregano
- For the dressing:
- ½ cup mayonnaise
- 2 tablespoons grated Parmesan cheese
- 2 tablespoons freshly squeezed lemon juice
- 1 clove garlic, peeled and smashed
- 1 teaspoon Dijon mustard
- ½ tablespoon Worcestershire sauce
- ½ tablespoon anchovy paste
- For the salad:
- 3 heads romaine lettuce, cut into bite-size pieces

DIRECTIONS:
1. Preheat the oven to 450°F. Line a baking sheet with parchment paper. In a medium bowl, toss together the chickpeas, oil, salt, garlic powder, onion powder, and oregano.

2. Scatter the coated chickpeas on the prepared baking sheet. Roast for about 20 minutes, tossing occasionally, until the chickpeas are golden and have a bit of crunch.
3. In a small bowl, whisk the mayonnaise, Parmesan, lemon juice, garlic, mustard, Worcestershire sauce, and anchovy paste until combined.
4. In a large bowl, combine the lettuce and dressing. Toss to coat. Top with the roasted chickpeas and serve.

NUTRITION: Calories: 367 Fat: 22g Carbs: 35g Protein: 12g

Coleslaw Worth A Second Helping

Preparation Time : 20 minutes

Cooking Time: 10 minutes

Servings: 6

INGREDIENTS:
- 5 cups shredded cabbage
- 2 carrots, shredded
- 1/3 cup chopped fresh flat-leaf parsley
- ½ cup mayonnaise
- ½ cup sour cream
- 3 tablespoons apple cider vinegar
- 1 teaspoon kosher salt
- ½ teaspoon celery seed

DIRECTIONS:
1. In a large bowl, combine the cabbage, carrots, and parsley. In a small bowl, whisk the mayonnaise, sour cream, vinegar, salt, and celery seed until smooth.
2. Pour the dressing over the vegetables and toss until coated. Transfer to a serving bowl and chill until ready to serve.

NUTRITION: Calories: 192 Fat: 18g Carbs: 7g Protein: 2g

Romaine Lettuce and Radicchios Mix

Preparation Time: 6 minutes

Cooking Time: 0 minutes

Servings: 4

INGREDIENTS:
- 2 tablespoons olive oil
- A pinch of salt and black pepper
- 2 spring onions, chopped
- 3 tablespoons Dijon mustard
- Juice of 1 lime
- ½ cup basil, chopped
- 4 cups romaine lettuce heads, chopped
- 3 radicchios, sliced

DIRECTIONS:
1. In a salad bowl, mix the lettuce with the spring onions and the other ingredients, toss and serve.

NUTRITION: Calories: 87 Fats: 2 g Carbs: 1 g Protein: 2 g

Asparagus and Smoked Salmon Salad

Preparation Time: 15 minutes
Cooking Time : 10 minutes

Servings: 8

INGREDIENTS:
- 1 lb. fresh asparagus, trimmed and cut into 1-inch pieces
- 1/2 cup pecans,
- 2 heads red leaf lettuce, rinsed and torn
- 1/2 cup frozen green peas, thawed
- 1/4 lb. smoked salmon, cut into 1-inch chunks
- 1/4 cup olive oil
- 2 tablespoons. lemon juice
- 1 teaspoon Dijon mustard
- 1/2 teaspoon salt
- 1/4 teaspoon pepper

DIRECTIONS:
2. Boil a pot of water. Stir in asparagus and cook for 5 minutes until tender. Let it drain; set aside. In a skillet, cook the pecans over medium heat for 5 minutes, stirring constantly until lightly toasted.
3. Combine the asparagus, toasted pecans, salmon, peas, and red leaf lettuce and toss in a large bowl.
4. In another bowl, combine lemon juice, pepper, Dijon mustard, salt, and olive oil. You can coat the salad with the dressing or serve it on its side.

NUTRITION: Calories: 159 Carbohydrate: 7 g Fat: 12.9 g Protein: 6 g

Shrimp Cobb Salad

Preparation Time : 25 minutes
Cooking Time : 10 minutes

Servings: 2

INGREDIENTS:
- 4 slices center-cut bacon
- 1 lb. large shrimp, peeled and deveined
- 1/2 teaspoon ground paprika
- 1/4 teaspoon ground black pepper
- 1/4 teaspoon salt, divided
- 2 1/2 tablespoons. Fresh lemon juice
- 1 1/2 tablespoons. Extra-virgin olive oil
- 1/2 teaspoon whole grain Dijon mustard
- 1 (10 oz.) package romaine lettuce hearts, chopped
- 2 cups cherry tomatoes, quartered
- 1 ripe avocado, cut into wedges
- 1 cup shredded carrots

DIRECTIONS:
1. In a large skillet over medium heat, cook the bacon for 4 minutes on each side till crispy. Take away from the skillet and place on paper towels; let cool for 5 minutes. Break the bacon into bits.
2. Pour out most of the bacon fat, leaving behind only 1 tablespoon. in the skillet. Bring the skillet back to medium-high heat.
3. Add black pepper and paprika to the shrimp for seasoning. Cook the shrimp around 2 minutes each side until it is opaque. Sprinkle with 1/8 teaspoon of salt for seasoning.

4. Combine the remaining 1/8 teaspoon of salt, mustard, olive oil and lemon juice together in a small bowl. Stir in the romaine hearts.
5. On each serving plate, place on 1 and 1/2 cups of romaine lettuce. Add on top the same amounts of avocado, carrots, tomatoes, shrimp and bacon.

NUTRITION: Calories: 528 Carbohydrate: 22.7 g Fat: 28.7 g Protein: 48.9 g

Classic Niçoise Salad

Preparation time : 15 minutes

Cooking time: 15 minutes

Servings: 4

INGREDIENTS:
- 1-pound red potatoes, cut into 1-inch pieces
- 4 tablespoons white wine vinegar, divided
- 8 ounces green beans, trimmed
- ¼ cup extra-virgin olive oil
- 1 teaspoon Dijon mustard
- 1 teaspoon fresh thyme leaves
- ½ teaspoon salt
- ¼ teaspoon freshly ground black pepper
- 1 head butter lettuce, chopped
- 1 (5-ounce) can tuna in olive oil, drained
- ½ cup pitted Niçoise olives
- 1/3 cup chopped tomato
- 2 scallions, chopped
- 4 large eggs, hard-boiled, peeled, and sliced

DIRECTIONS:
1. Put the potatoes in a saucepan, cover with water, and bring to a boil over high heat. Cook for about 10 minutes, until tender. Drain and transfer to a bowl. Sprinkle with 1 tablespoon of vinegar and let sit.
2. While the potatoes are cooling, fill the same saucepan with water and bring to a boil over high heat. Fill a large bowl with ice cubes and water.

3. Add the green beans to the boiling water and blanch for 3 minutes, then remove with tongs or a strainer and immediately plunge them into the ice bath. Once cool, drain.
4. In a small bowl, whisk together the olive oil, remaining 3 tablespoons of vinegar, mustard, thyme, salt, and pepper.
5. In a large bowl, combine the lettuce, tuna, olives, tomato, and scallions. Add half of the dressing and toss to coat.
6. Arrange the lettuce mixture on serving plates. Divide the potatoes, green beans, and eggs on top. Drizzle with the remaining dressing.

NUTRITION: Calories: 373 Fat: 23g Protein: 18g Carbohydrates: 25g

Algerian Carrot Slaw

Preparation time: 50 minutes

Cooking time: 0 minutes

Servings: 6

INGREDIENTS:
- ¼ cup extra-virgin olive oil
- Juice of ½ lemon
- 2 tablespoons cider vinegar
- ½ teaspoon salt
- ¼ teaspoon freshly ground black pepper
- Pinch smoked paprika
- Pinch red pepper flakes (optional)
- 1-pound carrots, shredded
- 2 fennel bulbs, trimmed and shredded
- 1/3 cup chopped pitted olives
- 1/3 cup thinly sliced oil-packed sun-dried tomatoes
- ¼ cup chopped fresh flat-leaf parsley

DIRECTIONS:
1. In a small bowl, whisk together the olive oil, lemon juice, vinegar, salt, black pepper, paprika, and red pepper flakes (if using).
2. In a large bowl, combine the carrots, fennel, olives, and sun-dried tomatoes. Add the dressing and toss well to coat. Chill for 30 minutes, then garnish with the parsley.

NUTRITION: Calories: 159 Fat: 11g Protein: 2g Carbohydrates: 15g

Tabbouleh (Lebanese Parsley and Bulgur Salad)

Preparation time: 15 minutes

Cooking time: 20 minutes

Servings: 4

INGREDIENTS:
- 1 cup bulgur
- 4 plum tomatoes, diced, juices reserved
- 2 cups finely chopped fresh flat-leaf parsley
- 4 scallions, chopped
- ¼ cup extra-virgin olive oil
- Juice of 2 lemons
- 2 tablespoons finely chopped fresh mint
- ½ teaspoon salt
- ¼ teaspoon freshly ground black pepper

DIRECTIONS:
1. In a saucepan, prepare the bulgur according to package directions. Drain thoroughly, transfer to a large bowl, and set aside to cool. Once cool, add the tomatoes with their juices, parsley, and scallions.
2. In a small bowl, whisk together the olive oil, lemon juice, mint, salt, and pepper. Pour the dressing over the bulgur mixture and toss to coat.

NUTRITION: Calories: 271 Fat: 14g Protein: 6g Carbohydrates: 34g

Cucumber and Red Onion Salad

Preparation time: 15 minutes

Cooking time: 0 minutes

Servings: 4

INGREDIENTS:
- ¼ cup extra-virgin olive oil
- 1 tablespoon red wine vinegar
- 1 teaspoon dried oregano
- Pinch salt
- Freshly ground black pepper
- 2 cucumbers, peeled and sliced
- ½ red onion, thinly sliced

DIRECTIONS:
1. In a small bowl, whisk together the olive oil, vinegar, and oregano. Season with the salt and pepper to taste.
2. In a bowl, combine the cucumbers and red onion. Add the dressing and toss well to coat.

NUTRITION: Calories: 143 Fat: 14g Protein: 1g Carbohydrates: 4g

Mediterranean Quinoa Salad

Preparation time: 15 minutes

Cooking time: 15 minutes

Servings: 4

INGREDIENTS:
- 1½ cups quinoa
- 2 cucumbers, seeded and diced
- 1 small red onion, diced
- 1 large tomato, diced
- 1 handful fresh flat-leaf parsley, chopped
- ½ cup extra-virgin olive oil
- ¼ cup red wine vinegar
- Juice of 1 lemon
- 1½ teaspoons salt
- ¾ teaspoon freshly ground black pepper
- 4 heads endive, trimmed and separated into spears
- 1 avocado, pitted, peeled, and diced

DIRECTIONS:
1. In a saucepan, prepare the quinoa according to package directions. Rinse the quinoa under cold running water and drain very well. Transfer to a large bowl. Add the cucumbers, red onion, tomato, and parsley.
2. In a small bowl, whisk together the olive oil, vinegar, lemon juice, salt, and pepper. Pour the dressing over the quinoa mixture and toss to coat. Spoon the mixture onto the endive spears and top with the

avocado.
NUTRITION: Calories: 669 Fat: 40g Protein: 17g Carbohydrates: 69g

French Potato Dijon Herb Salad

Preparation time: 15 minutes

Cooking time: 10 minutes

Servings: 4-6

INGREDIENTS:
- ¼ cup extra-virgin olive oil
- ½ teaspoon pepper
- 1 garlic clove, peeled and threaded on skewer
- 1 small shallot, minced
- 1 tablespoon minced fresh chervil
- 1 tablespoon minced fresh chives
- 1 tablespoon minced fresh parsley
- 1 teaspoon minced fresh tarragon
- 1½ tablespoons white wine vinegar or Champagne vinegar
- 2 pounds small red potatoes, unpeeled, sliced ¼ inch thick
- 2 tablespoons salt
- 2 teaspoons Dijon mustard

DIRECTIONS:
1. Place potatoes in a big saucepan, put in water to cover by 1 inch, and bring to boil on high heat. Put in salt, decrease the heat to simmer, and cook until potatoes are soft and paring knife can be slipped in and out of potatoes with little resistance, about 6 minutes.
2. While potatoes are cooking, lower skewered garlic into simmering water and

blanch for 45 seconds. Run garlic under cold running water, then remove from skewer and mince.
3. Reserve ¼ cup cooking water, then drain potatoes and lay out on tight one layer in rimmed baking sheet.
4. Beat oil, minced garlic, vinegar, mustard, pepper, and reserved potato cooking water together in a container, then drizzle over potatoes. Let potatoes sit until flavors blend, about 10 minutes.
5. Move potatoes to big container. Mix shallot and herbs in a small-sized container, then drizzle over potatoes and gently toss to coat using rubber spatula. Serve.

NUTRITION: Calories: 140 Carbs: 1g Fat: 15g Protein: 1g

Green Bean Cilantro Salad

Preparation time: 15 minutes

Cooking time: 15 minutes

Servings: 6-8

INGREDIENTS:
- ¼ cup walnuts
- ½ cup extra-virgin olive oil
- 1 scallion, sliced thin
- 2 garlic cloves, unpeeled
- 2 pounds green beans, trimmed
- 2½ cups fresh cilantro leaves and stems, tough stem ends trimmed (about 2 bunches)
- 4 teaspoons lemon juice
- Salt and pepper

DIRECTIONS:
1. Cook walnuts and garlic in 8-inch frying pan on moderate heat, stirring frequently, until toasted and aromatic, 5 to 7 minutes; move to a container. Let garlic cool slightly, then peel and approximately chop.
2. Process walnuts, garlic, cilantro, oil, lemon juice, scallion, ½ teaspoon salt, and 1/8 teaspoon pepper using a food processor until smooth, about 1 minute, scraping down sides of the container as required; move to big container.
3. Bring 4 quarts water to boil in large pot on high heat. In the meantime, fill big container halfway with ice and water.

4. Put in 1 tablespoon salt and green beans to boiling water and cook until crisp-tender, 3 to 5 minutes. Drain green beans, move to ice water, and allow to sit until chilled, approximately two minutes.
5. Move green beans to a container with cilantro sauce and gently toss until coated. Sprinkle with salt and pepper to taste. Serve.

NUTRITION: Calories: 145 Carbs: 0g Fat: 8g Protein: 0g

Italian Panzanella Mix Salad

Preparation time : 15 minutes

Cooking time: 20 minutes

Servings: 6

INGREDIENTS:
- 1 (15-ounce) can cannellini beans, rinsed
- 1 small red onion, halved and sliced thin
- 1½ pounds ripe tomatoes, cored and chopped, seeds and juice reserved
- 12 ounces rustic Italian bread, cut into 1-inch pieces (4 cups)
- 2 ounces Parmesan cheese, shaved
- 2 tablespoons minced fresh oregano
- 3 ounces (3 cups) baby arugula
- 3 tablespoons chopped fresh basil
- 3 tablespoons red wine vinegar
- 5 tablespoons extra-virgin olive oil
- Salt and pepper

DIRECTIONS:
1. Place the oven rack in the center of the oven and pre-heat your oven to 350 degrees. Toss bread pieces with 1 tablespoon oil and sprinkle with salt and pepper.
2. Arrange bread in one layer in rimmed baking sheet and bake, stirring intermittently, until light golden brown, fifteen to twenty minutes. Allow it to cool to room temperature.

3. Beat vinegar and ¼ teaspoon salt together in a big container. Whisking continuously, slowly drizzle in remaining ¼ cup oil.
4. Put in tomatoes with their seeds and juice, beans, onion, 1½ tablespoons basil, and 1 tablespoon oregano, toss to coat, and allow to sit for 20 minutes.
5. Put in cooled croutons, arugula, remaining 1½ tablespoons basil, and remaining 1 tablespoon oregano and gently toss to combine.
6. Sprinkle with salt and pepper to taste. Move salad to serving platter and drizzle with Parmesan. Serve.

NUTRITION: Calories: 294 Carbs: 32g Fat: 15g Protein: 9g

Mackerel-Fennel-Apple Salad

Preparation time: 15 minutes

Cooking time: 0 minutes

Servings: 4-6

INGREDIENTS:
- ¼ cup extra-virgin olive oil
- 1 fennel bulb, stalks discarded, bulb halved, cored, and sliced thin
- 1 small shallot, minced
- 1 tablespoon whole-grain mustard
- 2 Granny Smith apples, peeled, cored, and cut into 3-inch-long matchsticks
- 2 teaspoons minced fresh tarragon
- 3 tablespoons lemon juice
- 5 ounces (5 cups) watercress
- 6 ounces smoked mackerel, skin and pin bones removed, flaked
- Salt and pepper

DIRECTIONS:
1. Beat lemon juice, mustard, shallot, 1 teaspoon tarragon, ½ teaspoon salt, and ¼ teaspoon pepper together in a big container.
2. Whisking continuously, slowly drizzle in oil. Put in watercress, apples, and fennel and gently toss to coat. Sprinkle with salt and pepper to taste.
3. Divide salad among plates and top with flaked mackerel. Sprinkle any remaining dressing over mackerel and drizzle with

remaining 1 teaspoon tarragon. Serve instantly.

NUTRITION: Calories: 157 Carbs: 12g Fat: 13g Protein: 1g

Moroccan Carrot Salad

Preparation time: 15 minutes

Cooking time: 0 minutes

Servings: 4-6

INGREDIENTS:
- 1/8 teaspoon cayenne pepper
- 1/8 teaspoon ground cinnamon
- ¾ teaspoon ground cumin
- 1-pound carrots, peeled and shredded
- 1 tablespoon lemon juice
- 1 teaspoon honey
- 2 oranges
- 3 tablespoons extra-virgin olive oil
- 3 tablespoons minced fresh cilantro
- Salt and pepper

DIRECTIONS:
1. Cut away peel and pith from oranges. Holding fruit over bowl, use paring knife to slice between membranes to release segments.
2. Cut segments in half crosswise and allow to drain in fine-mesh strainer set over big container, reserving juice.
3. Beat lemon juice, honey, cumin, cayenne, cinnamon, and ½ teaspoon salt into reserved orange juice.
4. Put in drained oranges and carrots and gently toss to coat. Allow to sit until liquid starts to pool in bottom of bowl, 3 to 5 minutes.

5. Drain salad in fine-mesh strainer and return to now-empty bowl. Mix in cilantro and oil and sprinkle with salt and pepper to taste. Serve.

NUTRITION: Calories: 84 Carbs: 13g Fat: 4g Protein: 1g

Algerian Mix Salad

Preparation time: 15 minutes

Cooking time: 0 minutes

Servings: 4-6

INGREDIENTS:
- ¼ cup coarsely chopped fresh mint
- ¼ cup extra-virgin olive oil
- ½ cup pitted oil-cured black olives, quartered
- 2 fennel bulbs, stalks discarded, bulbs halved, cored, and sliced thin
- 2 tablespoons lemon juice
- 4 blood oranges
- Salt and pepper

DIRECTIONS:
1. Cut away peel and pith from oranges. Quarter oranges, then slice crosswise into ¼-inch-thick pieces. Mix oranges, fennel, olives, and mint in a big container.
2. Beat lemon juice, ¼ teaspoon salt, and 1/8 teaspoon pepper together in a small-sized container. Whisking continuously, slowly drizzle in oil.
3. Sprinkle dressing over salad and gently toss to coat. Sprinkle with salt and pepper to taste. Serve.

NUTRITION: Calories: 180 Carbs: 21g Fat: 11g Protein: 3g

Asparagus Mix Salad

Preparation time: 15 minutes

Cooking time: 0 minutes

Servings: 4-6

INGREDIENTS:
- Pesto:
- ¼ cup fresh basil leaves
- ¼ cup grated Pecorino Romano cheese
- ½ cup extra-virgin olive oil
- 1 garlic clove, minced
- 1 teaspoon grated lemon zest plus 2 teaspoons juice
- 2 cups fresh mint leaves
- Salt and pepper
- Salad:
- ¾ cup hazelnuts, toasted, skinned, and chopped
- 2 oranges
- 2 pounds asparagus, trimmed
- 4 ounces feta cheese, crumbled (1 cup)
- Salt and pepper

DIRECTIONS:
1. For the Pesto, process mint, basil, Pecorino, lemon zest and juice, garlic, and ¾ teaspoon salt using a food processor until finely chopped, approximately half a minute, scraping down sides of the container as required. Move to big container. Mix in oil and sprinkle with salt and pepper to taste.

2. For the Salad, chop asparagus tips from stalks into ¾-inch-long pieces. Cut asparagus stalks 1/8 inch thick on bias into approximate 2-inch lengths.
3. Cut away the peel and pith from oranges. Holding fruit over bowl, use paring knife to cut between membranes to release segments.
4. Put in asparagus tips and stalks, orange segments, feta, and hazelnuts to pesto and toss to combine. Sprinkle with salt and pepper to taste. Serve.

NUTRITION: Calories: 220 Carbs: 40g Fat: 5g Protein: 6g

Brussels Pecorino Pine Salad

Preparation time: 15 minutes

Cooking time: 0 minutes

Servings: 4-6

INGREDIENTS:
- ¼ cup extra-virgin olive oil
- ¼ cup pine nuts, toasted
- 1 garlic clove, minced
- 1 pound Brussels sprouts, trimmed, halved, and sliced very thin
- 1 small shallot, minced
- 1 tablespoon Dijon mustard
- 2 ounces Pecorino Romano cheese, shredded (2/3 cup)
- 2 tablespoons lemon juice
- Salt and pepper

DIRECTIONS:
1. Beat lemon juice, mustard, shallot, garlic, and ½ teaspoon salt together in a big container. Whisking continuously, slowly drizzle in oil.
2. Put in Brussels sprouts, toss to coat, and allow to sit for minimum half an hour or maximum 2 hours. Mix in Pecorino and pine nuts. Sprinkle with salt and pepper to taste. Serve.

NUTRITION: Calories: 353 Carbs: 37g Fat: 16g Protein: 13g

Cauliflower Chermoula Salad

Preparation time: 15 minutes

Cooking time: 22 minutes

Servings: 4-6

INGREDIENTS:
- Salad:
- ½ cup raisins
- ½ red onion, sliced ¼ inch thick
- 1 cup shredded carrot
- 1 head cauliflower (2 pounds), cored and cut into 2-inch florets
- 2 tablespoons chopped fresh cilantro
- 2 tablespoons extra-virgin olive oil
- 2 tablespoons sliced almonds, toasted
- Salt and pepper
- Chermoula:
- 1/8 teaspoon cayenne pepper
- ¼ cup extra-virgin olive oil
- ¼ teaspoon salt
- ½ teaspoon ground cumin
- ½ teaspoon paprika
- ¾ cup fresh cilantro leaves
- 2 tablespoons lemon juice
- 4 garlic cloves, minced

DIRECTIONS:
1. For the salad, place oven rack to lowest position and pre-heat your oven to 475 degrees. Toss cauliflower with oil and sprinkle with salt and pepper.

2. Arrange cauliflower in one layer in parchment paper–lined rimmed baking sheet. Cover tightly with aluminum foil and roast till they become tender, 5 to 7 minutes.
3. Remove foil and spread onion evenly in sheet. Roast until vegetables are tender, cauliflower becomes deeply golden brown, and onion slices are charred at edges, 10 to 15 minutes, stirring halfway through roasting. Allow it to cool slightly, approximately five minutes.
4. For the chermoula, process all ingredients using a food processor until smooth, about 1 minute, scraping down sides of the container as required. Move to big container.
5. Gently toss cauliflower-onion mixture, carrot, raisins, and cilantro with chermoula until coated. Move to serving platter and drizzle with almonds. Serve warm or at room temperature.

NUTRITION: Calories: 450 Carbs: 77g Fat: 7g Protein: 20g

Cherry Tomato Mix Salad

Preparation time: 15 minutes

Cooking time: 10 minutes

Servings: 4-6

INGREDIENTS:
- ½ cup pitted kalamata olives, chopped
- ½ teaspoon sugar
- 1 shallot, minced
- 1 small cucumber, peeled, halved along the length, seeded, and cut into ½-inch pieces
- 1 tablespoon red wine vinegar
- 1½ pounds cherry tomatoes, quartered
- 2 garlic cloves, minced
- 2 tablespoons extra-virgin olive oil
- 2 teaspoons minced fresh oregano
- 3 tablespoons chopped fresh parsley
- 4 ounces feta cheese, crumbled (1 cup)
- Salt and pepper

DIRECTIONS:
1. Toss tomatoes with sugar and ¼ teaspoon salt in a container and allow to sit for 30 minutes.
2. Move tomatoes to salad spinner and spin until seeds and excess liquid have been removed, 45 to 60 seconds, stopping to redistribute tomatoes several times during spinning.
3. Put in tomatoes, cucumber, olives, feta, and parsley to big container; set aside.
4. Strain ½ cup tomato liquid through fine-mesh strainer into liquid measuring cup;

discard remaining liquid.
5. Bring tomato liquid, shallot, vinegar, garlic, and oregano to simmer in small saucepan on moderate heat and cook until reduced to 3 tablespoons, 6 to 8 minutes.
6. Move to small-sized container and allow to cool to room temperature, approximately five minutes. Whisking continuously, slowly drizzle in oil.
7. Sprinkle dressing over salad and gently toss to coat. Sprinkle with salt and pepper to taste. Serve.

NUTRITION: Calories: 110 Carbs: 20g Fat: 4g Protein: 1g

Classic Greek Salad

Preparation time: 15 minutes

Cooking time: 0 minutes

Servings : 6-8

INGREDIENTS:
- ¼ cup chopped fresh mint
- ¼ cup chopped fresh parsley
- ½ cup pitted kalamata olives, quartered
- ½ red onion, sliced thin
- 1 cup jarred roasted red peppers, rinsed, patted dry, and cut into ½-inch strips
- 1 garlic clove, minced
- 1 teaspoon lemon juice
- 1½ tablespoons red wine vinegar
- 2 cucumbers, peeled, halved along the length, seeded, and sliced thin
- 2 teaspoons minced fresh oregano
- 5 ounces feta cheese, crumbled (1¼ cups)
- 6 large ripe tomatoes, cored, seeded, and cut into ½-inch-thick wedges
- 6 tablespoons extra-virgin olive oil
- Salt and pepper

DIRECTIONS:
1. Beat oil, vinegar, oregano, lemon juice, garlic, ½ teaspoon salt, and 1/8 teaspoon pepper together in a big container. Put in cucumbers and onion, toss to coat, and allow to sit for 20 minutes.
2. Put in tomatoes, red peppers, olives, parsley, and mint to a container with cucumber-onion mixture and toss to

combine.
3. Sprinkle with salt and pepper to taste. Move salad to wide, shallow serving bowl or platter and drizzle with feta. Serve instantly.

NUTRITION: Calories: 100 Carbs: 5g Fat: 8g Protein: 2g

Crunchy Mushroom Salad

Preparation time: 15 minutes
Cooking time : 0 minutes

Servings: 6

INGREDIENTS:
- ¼ cup extra-virgin olive oil
- ½ cup fresh parsley leaves
- 1 shallot, halved and sliced thin
- 1½ tablespoons lemon juice
- 2 ounces Parmesan cheese, shaved
- 2 tablespoons chopped fresh tarragon
- 4 celery ribs, sliced thin, plus ½ cup celery leaves
- 8 ounces cremini mushrooms, trimmed and sliced thin
- Salt and pepper

DIRECTIONS:
1. Beat oil, lemon juice, and ¼ teaspoon salt together in a big container. Put in mushrooms and shallot, toss to coat, and allow to sit for about ten minutes.
2. Put in sliced celery and leaves, Parmesan, parsley, and tarragon to mushroom-shallot mixture and toss to combine. Sprinkle with salt and pepper to taste. Serve.

NUTRITION: Calories: 70 Carbs: 1g Fat: 3g Protein: 1g

Cucumber Sesame-Lemon Salad

Preparation time: 1-3 hours & 15 minutes

Cooking time: 0 minutes

Servings: 4

INGREDIENTS:
- 1/8 teaspoon red pepper flakes, plus extra for seasoning
- ¼ cup rice vinegar
- 1 tablespoon lemon juice
- 1 tablespoon sesame seeds, toasted
- 2 tablespoons toasted sesame oil
- 2 teaspoons sugar
- 3 cucumbers, peeled, halved along the length, seeded, and sliced ¼ inch thick
- Salt and pepper

DIRECTIONS:
1. Toss cucumbers with 1 tablespoon salt using a colander set over big container. Weight cucumbers with 1 gallon-size zipper-lock bag filled with water; drain for 1 to three hours. Wash and pat dry.
2. Beat vinegar, oil, lemon juice, sesame seeds, sugar, and pepper flakes together in a big container. Put in cucumbers and toss to coat. Sprinkle with salt and pepper to taste. Serve at room temperature or chilled.

NUTRITION: Calories: 187 Carbs: 29g Fat: 7g Protein: 6g

Cut Up Salad

Preparation time: 15 minutes

Cooking time: 0 minutes

Servings: 4

INGREDIENTS:
- ½ cup chopped fresh parsley
- ½ cup pitted kalamata olives, chopped
- ½ small red onion, chopped fine
- 1 (15-ounce) can chickpeas, rinsed
- 1 cucumber, peeled, halved along the length, seeded, and cut into ½-inch pieces
- 1 garlic clove, minced
- 1 romaine lettuce heart (6 ounces), cut into ½-inch pieces
- 10 ounces grape tomatoes, quartered
- 3 tablespoons extra-virgin olive oil
- 3 tablespoons red wine vinegar
- 4 ounces feta cheese, crumbled (1 cup)
- Salt and pepper

DIRECTIONS:
1. Toss cucumber and tomatoes with 1 teaspoon salt and allow to drain using a colander for about fifteen minutes.
2. Beat vinegar and garlic together in a big container. Whisking continuously, slowly drizzle in oil.
3. Put in cucumber-tomato mixture, chickpeas, olives, onion, and parsley and toss to coat. Allow to sit for minimum 5 minutes or maximum 20 minutes.

4. Put in lettuce and feta and gently toss to combine. Sprinkle with salt and pepper to taste. Serve.

NUTRITION: Calories: 170 Carbs: 0g Fat: 8g Protein: 22g

Fattoush

Preparation time: 15 minutes

Cooking time: 15 minutes

Servings: 4-6

INGREDIENTS:
- ¼ teaspoon minced garlic
- ½ cup chopped fresh cilantro
- ½ cup chopped fresh mint
- 1 cup arugula, chopped coarse
- 1 English cucumber, peeled and sliced 1/8 inch thick
- 1-pound ripe tomatoes, cored and cut into ¾-inch pieces
- 2 (8-inch) pita breads
- 3 tablespoons lemon juice
- 4 scallions, sliced thin
- 4 teaspoons ground sumac, plus extra for sprinkling
- 7 tablespoons extra-virgin olive oil
- Salt and pepper

DIRECTIONS:
1. Place the oven rack in the center of the oven and pre-heat your oven to 375 degrees. Using kitchen shears, slice around perimeter of each pita and divide into 2 thin rounds.
2. Cut each round in half. Place pitas smooth side down on wire rack set in rimmed baking sheet. Brush 3 tablespoons oil on surface of pitas.

3. Sprinkle with salt and pepper. Bake until pitas are crisp and pale golden brown, 10 to 14 minutes. Allow it to cool to room temperature.
4. Beat lemon juice, sumac, garlic, and ¼ teaspoon salt together in a small-sized container and allow to sit for about ten minutes. Whisking continuously, slowly drizzle in remaining ¼ cup oil.
5. Break pitas into ½-inch pieces and place in a big container. Put in tomatoes, cucumber, arugula, cilantro, mint, and scallions.
6. Sprinkle dressing over salad and gently toss to coat. Sprinkle with salt and pepper to taste. Serve, sprinkling individual portions with extra sumac.

NUTRITION: Calories: 97 Carbs: 23g Fat: 0g Protein: 4g

Toast with Smoked Salmon, Herbed Cream Cheese, and Greens

Preparation Time: 10 minutes
Cooking Time : 5 minutes

Servings: 2

INGREDIENTS :
- For the herbed cream cheese:
- ¼ cup cream cheese, at room temperature
- 2 tablespoons chopped fresh flat-leaf parsley
- 2 tablespoons chopped fresh chives or sliced scallion
- ½ teaspoon garlic powder
- ¼ teaspoon kosher salt
- For the toast:
- 2 slices bread
- 4 ounces smoked salmon
- Small handful microgreens or sprouts
- 1 tablespoon capers, drained and rinsed
- ¼ small red onion, very thinly sliced

DIRECTIONS:
1. In a medium bowl, combine the cream cheese, parsley, chives, garlic powder, and salt. Using a fork, mix until combined. Chill until ready to use.
2. Toast the bread until golden. Spread the herbed cream cheese over each piece of toast, then top with the smoked salmon. Garnish with the microgreens, capers, and red onion.

NUTRITION: Calories: 194 Fat: 8g Carbs: 2g Protein: 12g

Crab Melt with Avocado and Egg

Preparation Time: 15 minutes

Cooking Time: 15 minutes

Servings: 2

INGREDIENTS:
- 2 English muffins, split
- 3 tablespoons butter, divided
- 2 tomatoes, cut into slices
- 1 (4-ounce) can lump crabmeat
- 6 ounces sliced or shredded cheddar cheese
- 4 large eggs
- Kosher salt
- 2 large avocados, halved, pitted, and cut into slices
- Microgreens, for garnish

DIRECTIONS:
1. Preheat the broiler. Toast the English muffin halves. Place the toasted halves, cut-side up, on a baking sheet. Spread 1½ teaspoons of butter evenly over each half, allowing the butter to melt into the crevices.
2. Top each with tomato slices, then divide the crab over each, and finish with the cheese. Broil for about 4 minutes until the cheese melts.
3. Meanwhile, in a medium skillet over medium heat, melt the remaining 1 tablespoon of butter, swirling to coat the

bottom of the skillet.
4. Crack the eggs into the skillet, giving ample space for each. Sprinkle with salt. Cook for about 3 minutes.
5. Flip the eggs and cook the other side until the yolks are set to your liking. Place 1 egg on each English muffin half. Top with avocado slices and microgreens.

NUTRITION: Calories: 1221 Fat: 84g Carbs: 2g Protein: 12g

Tomato Cucumber Avocado Salad

Preparation Time: 15 minutes

Cooking Time: 0 minutes

Servings: 4

INGREDIENTS:
- 12 oz cherry tomatoes, cut in half
- 5 small cucumbers, chopped
- 3 small avocados, chopped
- ½ tsp ground black pepper
- 2 tbsp olive oil
- 2 tbsp fresh lemon juice
- ¼ cup fresh cilantro, chopped
- 1 tsp sea salt

DIRECTIONS:
1. Add cherry tomatoes, cucumbers, avocados, and cilantro into the large mixing bowl and mix well. Mix together olive oil, lemon juice, black pepper, and salt and pour over salad.
2. Toss well and serve immediately.

NUTRITION: Calories 442 Fat 31 g Carbs 30.3 g Protein 2 g

Healthy Broccoli Salad

Preparation Time: 25 minutes

Cooking Time: 0 minutes

Servings: 6

INGREDIENTS:
- 3 cups broccoli, chopped
- 1 tbsp apple cider vinegar
- ½ cup Greek yogurt
- 2 tbsp sunflower seeds
- 3 bacon slices, cooked and chopped
- 1/3 cup onion, sliced
- ¼ tsp stevia

DIRECTIONS:
1. In a mixing bowl, mix together broccoli, onion, and bacon. In a small bowl, mix together yogurt, vinegar, and stevia and pour over broccoli mixture. Stir to combine.
2. Sprinkle sunflower seeds on top of the salad. Store salad in the refrigerator for 30 minutes. Serve and enjoy.

NUTRITION: Calories 90 Fat 9 g Carbs 4 g Protein 2 g

Avocado Lime Shrimp Salad

Preparation Time: 15 minutes
Cooking Time : 0 minutes

Servings: 2

INGREDIENTS:
- 14 ounces of jumbo cooked shrimp, peeled and deveined; chopped
- 4 ½ ounces of avocado, diced
- 1 ½ cup of tomato, diced
- ¼ cup of chopped green onion
- ¼ cup of jalapeno with the seeds removed, diced fine
- 1 teaspoon of olive oil
- 2 tablespoons of lime juice
- 1/8 teaspoon of salt
- 1 tablespoon of chopped cilantro

DIRECTIONS:
1. Get a small bowl and combine green onion, olive oil, lime juice, pepper, a pinch of salt. Wait for about 5 minutes for all of them to marinate and mellow the flavor of the onion.
2. Get a large bowl and combined chopped shrimp, tomato, avocado, jalapeno. Combine all of the ingredients, add cilantro, and gently toss. Add pepper and salt as desired.

NUTRITION: Calories: 314 Protein,: 26g Carbs: 15g Fats: 9g

Grilled Mahi-Mahi with Jicama Slaw

Preparation Time: 20 minutes

Cooking Time: 10 minutes

Servings: 4

INGREDIENTS:
- 1 teaspoon each for pepper and salt, divided
- 1 tablespoon of lime juice, divided
- 2 tablespoon + 2 teaspoons of extra virgin olive oil
- 4 raw mahi-mahi fillets, which should be about 8 oz. each
- ½ cucumber which should be thinly cut into long strips (it should yield about 1 cup)
- 1 jicama, which should be thinly cut into long strips (it should yield about 3 cups)
- 1 cup of alfalfa sprouts
- 2 cups of coarsely chopped watercress

DIRECTIONS:
1. Combine ½ teaspoon of both pepper and salt, 1 teaspoon of lime juice, and 2 teaspoons of oil in a small bowl. Then brush the mahi-mahi fillets all through with the olive oil mixture.
2. Grill the mahi-mahi on medium-high heat until it becomes done in about 5 minutes, turn it to the other side, and let it be done for about 5 minutes.
3. For the slaw, combine the watercress, cucumber, jicama, and alfalfa sprouts in a

bowl. Now combine ½ teaspoon of both pepper and salt, 2 teaspoons of lime juice, and 2 tablespoons of extra virgin oil in a small bowl. Drizzle it over slaw and toss together to combine.
NUTRITION: Calories: 320 Protein: 44g Carbohydrate: 10g Fat: 11 g

Mediterranean Chicken Salad

Preparation Time: 5 minutes

Cooking Time: 25 minutes

Servings: 4

INGREDIENTS:
- For Chicken:
- 1 ¾ lb. boneless, skinless chicken breast
- ¼ teaspoon each of pepper and salt (or as desired)
- 1 ½ tablespoon of butter, melted
- For Mediterranean salad:
- 1 cup of sliced cucumber
- 6 cups of romaine lettuce, that is torn or roughly chopped
- 10 pitted Kalamata olives
- 1 pint of cherry tomatoes
- 1/3 cup of reduced-fat feta cheese
- ¼ teaspoon each of pepper and salt (or lesser)
- 1 small lemon juice (it should be about 2 tablespoons)

DIRECTIONS:
1. Preheat your oven or grill to about 350F. Season the chicken with salt, butter, and black pepper. Roast or grill chicken until it reaches an internal temperature of 1650F in about 25 minutes.
2. Once your chicken breasts are cooked, remove and keep aside to rest for about 5 minutes before you slice it.

3. Combine all the salad ingredients you have and toss everything together very well. Serve the chicken with Mediterranean salad.

NUTRITION: Calories: 340 Protein: 45g Carbohydrate: 9g Fat: 4 g

Shrimp Salad Cocktails

Preparation Time: 35 minutes
Cooking Time : 35 minutes

Servings: 8

INGREDIENTS:
- 2 cups mayonnaise
- 6 plum tomatoes, seeded and finely chopped
- 1/4 cup ketchup
- 1/4 cup lemon juice
- 2 cups seedless red and green grapes, halved
- 1 tablespoon. Worcestershire sauce
- 2 lbs. peeled and deveined cooked large shrimp
- 2 celery ribs, finely chopped
- 3 tablespoons. minced fresh tarragon or 3 teaspoon dried tarragon
- salt and 1/4 teaspoon pepper
- shredded 2 of cups romaine
- papaya or 1/2 cup peeled chopped mango
- parsley or minced chives

DIRECTIONS:
1. Combine Worcestershire sauce, lemon juice, ketchup and mayonnaise together in a small bowl. Combine pepper, salt, tarragon, celery and shrimp together in a large bowl.
2. Put in 1 cup of dressing toss well to coat. Scoop 1 tablespoon. of the dressing into 8 cocktail glasses.

3. Layer each glass with 1/4 cup of lettuce, followed by 1/2 cup of the shrimp mixture, 1/4 cup of grapes, 1/3 cup of tomatoes and finally 1 tablespoon. of mango.
4. Spread the remaining dressing over top; sprinkle chives on top. Serve immediately.

NUTRITION: Calories: 580 Carbohydrate: 16 g Fat: 46 g Protein: 24 g

Garlic Chive Cauliflower Mash

Preparation Time: 20 minutes

Cooking Time: 18 minutes

Servings: 5

INGREDIENTS:
- 4 cups cauliflower
- 1/3 cup vegetarian mayonnaise
- 1 garlic clove
- 1/2 teaspoon. kosher salt
- 1 tablespoon. water
- 1/8 teaspoon. pepper
- 1/4 teaspoon. lemon juice
- 1/2 teaspoon lemon zest
- 1 tablespoon Chives, minced

DIRECTIONS:
1. In a bowl that is save to microwave, add the cauliflower, mayo, garlic, water, and salt/pepper and mix until the cauliflower is well coated. Cook on high for 15-18 minutes, until the cauliflower is almost mushy.
2. Blend the mixture in a strong blender until completely smooth, adding a little more water if the mixture is too chunky. Season with the remaining ingredients and serve.

NUTRITION: Calories: 178 Carbohydrate: 14 g Fat: 18 g Protein: 2 g

Beet Greens with Pine Nuts Goat Cheese

Preparation Time: 25 minutes

Cooking Time: 15 minutes

Servings: 3

INGREDIENTS:
- 4 cups beet tops, washed and chopped roughly
- 1 teaspoon. EVOO
- 1 tablespoon. no sugar added balsamic vinegar
- 2 oz. crumbled dry goat cheese
- 2 tablespoons. Toasted pine nuts

DIRECTIONS:
1. Warm the oil in a pan, then cook the beet greens on medium high heat until they release their moisture. Let it cook until almost tender.
2. Flavor with salt and pepper and remove from heat. Toss the greens in a mixture of balsamic vinegar and olive oil, then top with the nuts and cheese. Serve warm.

NUTRITION: Calories: 215 Carbohydrate: 4 g Fat: 18 g Protein: 10 g

Kale Slaw and Strawberry Salad + Poppyseed Dressing

Preparation Time: 10 minutes

Cooking Time: 20 minutes

Servings: 2

INGREDIENTS:
- Chicken breast; 8 ounces; sliced and baked
- Kale; 1 cup; chopped
- Slaw mix; 1 cup (cabbage, broccoli slaw, carrots mixed)
- Slivered almonds; 1/4 cup
- Strawberries; 1 cup; sliced
- For the dressing:
- Light mayonnaise; 1 tablespoon
- Dijon mustard
- Olive oil; 1 tablespoon
- Apple cider vinegar; 1 tablespoon
- Lemon juice; 1/2 teaspoon
- 1 tablespoon of honey
- Onion powder; 1/4 teaspoon
- Garlic powder; 1/4 teaspoon
- Poppyseeds

DIRECTIONS:
1. Whisk the dressing ingredients together until well mixed, then leave to cool in the fridge. Slice the chicken breasts.
2. Divide 2 bowls of spinach, slaw, and strawberries. Cover with a sliced breast of chicken (4 oz. each), then scatter with

almonds. Divide the dressing between the two bowls and drizzle.
NUTRITION: Calories: 150 Carbs: 17g Fat: 1g Protein: 7g

Spring Greek Salad

Preparation time: 15 minutes

Cooking time: 0 minutes

Servings: 4

INGREDIENTS:
- 1 head escarole, chopped
- 1 head curly chicory, chopped
- ¼ cup crumbled feta cheese
- ¼ cup pitted halved kalamata olives
- ¼ cup sliced seeded pepperoncini
- 3 tablespoons extra-virgin olive oil
- Juice of ½ lemon
- 2 garlic cloves, minced
- Pinch dried dill
- Salt
- Freshly ground black pepper

DIRECTIONS:
1. In a large bowl, toss together the escarole and chicory. Scatter the feta cheese, olives, and pepperoncini on top.
2. In a small bowl, whisk together the olive oil, lemon juice, and garlic. Season with the dill and salt and pepper to taste. Pour the dressing over the lettuce mixture and toss to combine.

NUTRITION: Calories: 173 Fat: 14g Protein: 5g Carbohydrates: 10g

Panzanella

Preparation time: 15 minutes

Cooking time: 10 minutes

Servings: 6

INGREDIENTS:
- ¼ cup extra-virgin olive oil, plus 3 tablespoons
- 6 stale hearty Italian bread slices, cut into cubes
- 6 tomatoes, cut into 1-inch pieces
- 1 cucumber, halved lengthwise and cut into half-moons
- 1 red bell pepper, seeded and finely chopped
- ½ onion, thinly sliced
- 2 tablespoons roughly chopped capers
- 2 tablespoons red wine vinegar
- 1 garlic clove, minced
- 1 teaspoon salt
- ¼ teaspoon freshly ground black pepper
- 1 teaspoon chopped fresh basil

DIRECTIONS:
1. In a large skillet, heat 3 tablespoons of olive oil over medium heat. Add the bread cubes and cook for about 10 minutes, until browned on all sides.
2. Transfer the bread cubes to a large bowl and add the tomatoes, cucumber, bell pepper, onion, and capers.
3. In a small bowl, whisk together the remaining ¼ cup of olive oil, the vinegar,

garlic, salt, and pepper. Pour the dressing over the salad and toss to combine well.
4. Let the salad rest for 30 minutes. Sprinkle the basil on top and serve.

NUTRITION: Calories: 205 Fat: 17g Protein: 3g Carbohydrates: 13g

Tuscan Tuna Salad

Preparation time: 15 minutes

Cooking time: 0 minutes

Servings: 4

INGREDIENTS:
- ¼ cup extra-virgin olive oil
- Juice of ½ lemon
- ½ teaspoon Dijon mustard
- Salt
- Freshly ground black pepper
- 2 (5-ounce) cans tuna in olive oil, drained
- 1 (19-ounce) can cannellini beans, rinsed and drained
- 12 marinated mushrooms, rinsed and halved if large
- 12 grape or cherry tomatoes, halved
- 1 or 2 celery stalks, sliced
- 1 teaspoon capers (optional)

DIRECTIONS:
1. In a small bowl, whisk together the olive oil, lemon juice, and mustard, and season with salt and pepper.
2. In a large bowl, combine the tuna, beans, mushrooms, tomatoes, celery, and capers (if using). Add the dressing and toss well. Season with additional salt and pepper, if desired.

NUTRITION: Calories: 389 Fat: 20g Protein: 26g Carbohydrates: 29g

Mediterranean Chopped Salad

Preparation time: 15 minutes

Cooking time: 20 minutes

Servings: 4

INGREDIENTS:
- 1 cup whole grains, such as red or white quinoa, millet, or buckwheat
- 1 (15-ounce) can chickpeas, rinsed and drained
- 2 cups baby spinach
- 1 cucumber, finely chopped
- ½ red bell pepper, finely chopped
- ½ fennel bulb, trimmed and finely chopped
- 1 celery stalk, finely chopped
- 1 carrot, finely chopped
- 1 plum tomato, finely chopped
- ½ red onion, finely chopped
- 1 cherry pepper, seeded and finely chopped
- ¼ cup extra-virgin olive oil
- 2 tablespoons white wine vinegar
- 1 teaspoon chopped fresh basil
- 1 garlic clove, minced
- Salt
- Freshly ground black pepper

DIRECTIONS:
1. Cook the whole grains according to package directions. Allow to cool. In a large bowl, toss the grains, chickpeas, spinach, cucumber, bell pepper, fennel, celery,

carrot, tomato, red onion, and cherry pepper.
2. In a small bowl, whisk together the olive oil, vinegar, basil, and garlic. Season with salt and pepper. Toss with the salad and serve.

NUTRITION: Calories: 401 Fat: 18g Protein: 12g Carbohydrates: 50g

Green Bean and Potato Salad

Preparation time : 15 minutes

Cooking time: 15 minutes

Servings: 4

INGREDIENTS:
- 2 russet potatoes, peeled and cut into 1-inch pieces
- 2 cups green beans, trimmed
- ¼ cup extra-virgin olive oil
- Juice of ½ lemon
- 1 teaspoon Italian Herb Blend
- 1 teaspoon salt
- ½ teaspoon freshly ground black pepper

DIRECTIONS:
1. Put the potatoes in a saucepan, cover with water, and bring to a boil over high heat. Cook for about 10 minutes, until tender. Drain and set aside to cool.
2. While the potatoes are cooling, fill the same saucepan with water and bring to a boil over high heat. Fill a large bowl with ice cubes and cold water.
3. Add the green beans to the boiling water and blanch for about 3 minutes, then remove with tongs or a sieve and immediately plunge them into the ice bath. Once cool, drain.
4. Combine the potatoes and green beans in a large bowl. Drizzle the olive oil over the vegetables and squeeze in the lemon juice.

Add the Italian herb blend, salt, and pepper and toss to combine.
NUTRITION: Calories: 282 Fat: 14g Protein: 5g Carbohydrates: 37g

Shrimp Salad

Preparation time: 15 minutes

Cooking time: 5 minutes

Servings: 4

INGREDIENTS:
- 1-pound large shrimp, peeled and deveined
- Juice of ½ lemon
- 2 celery stalks, chopped
- 3 scallions, chopped
- 1 garlic clove, minced
- Salt
- Freshly ground black pepper
- ½ cup vegan mayonnaise

DIRECTIONS:
1. Put the shrimp in a skillet and add a few tablespoons of water. Cook over medium heat for 2 to 3 minutes, until the shrimp turn pink. Drain and pat dry. Cut the shrimp into bite-size pieces and transfer a bowl.
2. Add the lemon juice and toss, then add the celery, scallions, and garlic. Season with salt and pepper. Toss again to combine. Add the vegan mayonnaise and fold gently to combine.

NUTRITION: Calories: 185 Fat: 11g Protein: 18g Carbohydrates: 4g

Warm Potato Salad

Preparation time : 15 minutes

Cooking time: 10 minutes

Servings: 4

INGREDIENTS:
- 6 red potatoes, cut into 1-inch pieces
- 1 tablespoon white wine vinegar
- 3 large eggs, hard-boiled, peeled, and chopped
- 2 celery stalks, finely chopped
- 1 small onion, finely chopped
- ½ cup mayonnaise or vegan mayonnaise
- 1 teaspoon Dijon mustard
- 1 teaspoon salt
- ¼ teaspoon freshly ground black pepper

DIRECTIONS:
1. Put the potatoes in a saucepan, cover with water, and bring to a boil over high heat. Cook for about 10 minutes, until tender. Drain and transfer to a large bowl, then sprinkle with the vinegar.
2. Add the eggs, celery, and onion and toss. Add the mayonnaise, mustard, salt, and pepper and toss to combine. Serve.

NUTRITION: Calories: 474 Fat: 25g Protein: 11g Carbohydrates: 53g

Summer Rainbow Salad

Preparation time: 15 minutes

Cooking time: 0 minutes

Servings: 4

INGREDIENTS:
- 1 cup chopped red or green leaf lettuce
- 1 cup chopped iceberg lettuce
- ½ cup baby arugula
- ½ cup chopped radicchio
- 1 cup mixed chopped or sliced vegetables, such as red cabbage, red onion, radish, red or yellow tomato, carrot, cucumber, and/or avocado
- ¼ cup extra-virgin olive oil
- Juice of ½ lemon
- ½ teaspoon salt
- ¼ teaspoon freshly ground black pepper
- ¼ teaspoon dried oregano

DIRECTIONS:
1. In a large salad bowl, combine the lettuces, arugula, radicchio, and mixed vegetables and gently toss.
2. In a small bowl, whisk together the olive oil, lemon juice, salt, pepper, and oregano. Pour the dressing over the salad and toss well to coat.

NUTRITION: Calories: 137 Fat: 14g Protein: 1g Carbohydrates: 4g

Arugula and White Bean Salad

Preparation time: 15 minutes

Cooking time: 0 minutes

Servings: 2

INGREDIENTS:
- 1 (15-ounce) can cannellini beans, rinsed and drained
- 2 cups baby arugula
- ¼ cup extra-virgin olive oil
- Juice of ½ lemon
- ½ teaspoon dried oregano
- ½ teaspoon salt
- ¼ teaspoon freshly ground black pepper
- 4 Italian seeded bread slices, toasted

DIRECTIONS:
1. In a medium bowl, combine the beans and arugula. In a small bowl, whisk together the olive oil, lemon juice, oregano, salt, and pepper. Pour over the salad and toss to coat.
2. To serve, spoon heaping portions of the salad over the toast.

NUTRITION: Calories: 469 Fat: 29g Protein: 14g Carbohydrates: 42g

Fennel and Orange Salad

Preparation time: 15 minutes

Cooking time: 0 minutes

Servings: 6

INGREDIENTS:
- 4 navel oranges, peeled, halved, and thinly sliced
- 3 fennel bulbs, trimmed and thinly sliced, fronds reserved for garnish
- 2 tablespoons extra-virgin olive oil
- 1 tablespoon white wine vinegar
- Salt
- Freshly ground black pepper

DIRECTIONS:
1. In a large bowl, combine the orange and fennel slices. In a small bowl, whisk together the olive oil and vinegar. Season with salt and pepper.
2. Pour the dressing over the orange and fennel and toss to combine. Roughly chop the fennel fronds and sprinkle them on top.

NUTRITION: Calories: 122 Fat: 5g Protein: 2g Carbohydrates: 20g

Balsamic Asparagus

Preparation time: 10 minutes

Cooking time: 15 minutes

Servings: 4

INGREDIENTS:
- 3 tablespoons olive oil
- 3 garlic cloves, minced
- 2 tablespoons shallot, chopped
- Salt and black pepper to the taste
- 2 teaspoons balsamic vinegar
- 1 and ½ pound asparagus, trimmed

DIRECTIONS:
1. Heat up a pan with the oil over medium-high heat, add the garlic and the shallot and sauté for 3 minutes.
2. Add the rest of the ingredients, cook for 12 minutes more, divide between plates and serve as a side dish.

NUTRITION: Calories 100 Fat 10.5g Carbs 2.3g Protein 2.1g

Lime Cucumber Mix

Preparation time: 10 minutes

Cooking time: 0 minutes

Servings : 8

INGREDIENTS:
- 4 cucumbers, chopped
- ½ cup green bell pepper, chopped
- 1 yellow onion, chopped
- 1 chili pepper, chopped
- 1 garlic clove, minced
- 1 teaspoon parsley, chopped
- 2 tablespoons lime juice
- 1 tablespoon dill, chopped
- Salt and black pepper to the taste
- 1 tablespoon olive oil

DIRECTIONS:
1. In a large bowl, mix the cucumber with the bell peppers and the rest of the ingredients, toss and serve as a side dish.

NUTRITION: Calories 123 Fat 4.3g Carbs 5.6g Protein 2g

Walnuts Cucumber Mix

Preparation time : 5 minutes

Cooking time: 0 minutes

Servings: 2

INGREDIENTS:
- 2 cucumbers, chopped
- 1 tablespoon olive oil
- Salt and black pepper to the taste
- 1 red chili pepper, dried
- 1 tablespoon lemon juice
- 3 tablespoons walnuts, chopped
- 1 tablespoon balsamic vinegar
- 1 teaspoon chives, chopped

DIRECTIONS:
1. In a bowl, mix the cucumbers with the oil and the rest of the ingredients, toss and serve as a side dish.

NUTRITION: Calories 121 Fat 2.3g Carbs 6.7g Protein 2.4g

Cheesy Beet Salad

Preparation time: 10 minutes

Cooking time: 1 hour

Servings: 4

INGREDIENTS:
- 4 beets, peeled and cut into wedges
- 3 tablespoons olive oil
- Salt and black pepper to the taste
- ¼ cup lime juice
- 8 slices goat cheese, crumbled
- 1/3 cup walnuts, chopped
- 1 tablespoon chive, chopped

DIRECTIONS:
1. In a roasting pan, combine the beets with the oil, salt and pepper, toss and bake at 400 degrees F for 1 hour.
2. Cool the beets down, transfer them to a bowl, add the rest of the ingredients, toss and serve as a side.

NUTRITION: Calories 156 Fat 4.2g Carbs 6.5g Protein 4g

Rosemary Beets

Preparation time: 10 minutes
Cooking time : 20 minutes

Servings: 4

INGREDIENTS:
- 4 medium beets, peeled and cubed
- 1/3 cup balsamic vinegar
- 1 teaspoon rosemary, chopped
- 1 garlic clove, minced
- ½ teaspoon Italian seasoning
- 1 tablespoon olive oil

DIRECTIONS:
1. Heat up a pan with the oil over medium heat, add the beets and the rest of the ingredients, toss, and cook for 20 minutes. Divide the mix between plates and serve as a side dish.

NUTRITION: Calories 165 Fat 3.4g Carbs 11.3g Protein 2.3g

Squash and Tomatoes Mix

Preparation time: 10 minutes

Cooking time: 20 minutes

Servings: 6

INGREDIENTS:
- 5 medium squash, cubed
- A pinch of salt and black pepper
- 3 tablespoons olive oil
- 1 cup pine nuts, toasted
- ¼ cup goat cheese, crumbled
- 6 tomatoes, cubed
- ½ yellow onion, chopped
- 2 tablespoons cilantro, chopped
- 2 tablespoons lemon juice

DIRECTIONS:
1. Heat up a pan with the oil over medium heat, add the onion and pine nuts and cook for 3 minutes.
2. Add the squash and the rest of the ingredients, cook everything for 15 minutes, divide between plates and serve as a side dish.

NUTRITION: Calories 200 Fat 4.5g Carbs 6.7g Protein 4g